THE HEALTHY GUT GUIDE

Nourish your body and boost your well-being from within.

JUDY KELLY

Contents

Introduction: The Gut-Health Connection

WELCOME TO The Healthy Gut Guide: Nourish Your Body and Boost Your Well-being from Within." In this transformative guide, we invite you to embark on a journey of discovery and explore the fascinating world of gut health. You are about to uncover the powerful link between your gut and your overall well-being, and learn how nourishing your gut can profoundly impact your physical, mental, and emotional health.

The human gut is an intricate ecosystem, home to trillions of microorganisms that form the gut microbiota. It plays a pivotal role in digestion, nutrient absorption, immune function, and even influences our mood and cognitive processes through the gut-brain axis. The health of our gut has far-reaching implications, extending beyond the confines of the digestive system.

In this book, we aim to demystify the complex relationship between your gut and your overall wellness. We will explore the signs and symptoms of an unhealthy gut, unravel the root causes of gut health disturbances, and provide you with practical strategies to nurture and heal your gut.

Nurturing your gut involves adopting a holistic approach that encompasses not only the foods you eat but also the way you live. We will delve into the importance of a balanced and diverse diet, highlighting gut-friendly foods and the benefits they offer. You will discover the incredible healing power of herbs and supplements that can support your gut health journey.

But gut health is not just about what you put into your body; it also involves the mind-body connection. We will explore the fascinating gut-brain axis and how our gut health influences our mental and emotional well-being. You will learn strategies to reduce stress, promote relaxation, and practice mindful eating, all of which contribute to gut and brain harmony.

Healing your gut is a critical aspect of this guide. We will delve into the concept of leaky gut syndrome and provide you with actionable steps to restore balance and repair damage. Through gut-healing protocols, dietary approaches, and lifestyle modifications, you will gain the tools to reclaim your gut health and optimize your overall well-being.

And it doesn't stop there. Gut health is important for individuals of all ages, from children to aging adults. We will explore the unique considerations and gut-friendly tips for supporting the health of your whole family, nurturing healthy habits that will benefit them throughout their lives.

In a world where modern living presents challenges to our gut health, we will guide you in maintaining your gut health in a changing environment. You will learn strategies to manage gut health while traveling, navigate the impact of technology on gut health, and sustain gut-friendly practices for lifelong well-being.

"The Healthy Gut Guide" is not just a book; it's an invitation to embrace a vibrantly healthy gut and unlock the tremendous potential it holds. Through knowledge, understanding, and actionable steps, you will gain the tools to nourish your body and boost your well-being from within. Get ready to embark on a transformative journey that will empower you to take control of your gut health and experience the profound benefits it offers.

So, let's delve into the remarkable world of gut health and begin your path to a happier, healthier you. Your gut awaits, ready to be nourished and nurtured. Get ready to unlock the secrets of "The Healthy Gut Guide: Nourish Your Body and Boost Your Well-being from Within."

Chapter 1: Understanding Your Gut: The Key to Total Wellness

The Role of the Gut in Overall Health

Our gut, often referred to as the "second brain," plays a crucial role in our overall health and well-being. Beyond its primary function of digesting and absorbing nutrients from the food we consume, the gut is home to trillions of microorganisms known as the gut microbiota. These microorganisms have a profound impact on various aspects of our health, from digestion and immune function to mental and emotional well-being. In this chapter, we will explore the vital role of the gut in overall health.

1. Digestion and Nutrient Absorption: The gut is responsible for breaking down the food we eat into smaller components and extracting essential nutrients that our body needs for optimal functioning. The lining of

the gut is equipped with specialized cells that facilitate the absorption of nutrients, such as vitamins, minerals, proteins, and fats. A healthy gut ensures efficient digestion and nutrient absorption, supporting our body's energy production, growth, and repair processes.

2. Gut Microbiota and Immune Function: The gut microbiota plays a critical role in the development and maintenance of a robust immune system. Beneficial bacteria in the gut help educate and train our immune system, ensuring it responds appropriately to harmful pathogens while tolerating harmless substances. A healthy gut microbiota helps protect against infections, supports the production of immune cells and antibodies, and promotes overall immune resilience.

3. Gut-Brain Axis and Mental Well-being: The gut and the brain are intricately connected through the gut-brain axis, a

bi-directional communication system. The gut microbiota produces neurotransmitters, such as serotonin, dopamine, and GABA, which play essential roles in regulating mood, emotions, and mental well-being. Disruptions in the gut microbiota can impact neurotransmitter production, potentially contributing to mood disorders, such as anxiety and depression.

4. Inflammation and Chronic Disease: The gut has a significant influence on systemic inflammation, which is at the root of many chronic diseases. An imbalanced gut microbiota, leaky gut syndrome (increased intestinal permeability), or chronic gut inflammation can trigger a cascade of inflammatory responses throughout the body. Chronic inflammation is associated with conditions such as cardiovascular disease, diabetes, autoimmune disorders, and even certain types of cancer.

5. Hormone Regulation: The gut plays a role in hormone regulation, including hormones involved in appetite control, metabolism, and satiety. Certain gut hormones, such as ghrelin and leptin, communicate with the brain to regulate hunger and fullness signals. Imbalances in the gut microbiota can disrupt this hormonal communication, potentially leading to weight imbalances and metabolic dysregulation.

6. Detoxification: The gut is responsible for eliminating toxins, waste products, and harmful substances from our body. A healthy gut ensures proper detoxification and elimination processes, preventing the accumulation of toxins that can negatively impact our health. The gut microbiota also plays a role in breaking down and metabolizing certain compounds, such as medications and environmental toxins.

7. Nutrient Production: The gut microbiota assists in the production of essential

nutrients, such as certain vitamins and short-chain fatty acids (SCFAs). These SCFAs provide energy for the cells lining the gut, support a healthy gut barrier, and have anti-inflammatory properties. Additionally, the gut microbiota can help convert dietary fibers into beneficial substances that nourish the gut and promote overall health.

Understanding the pivotal role of the gut in overall health highlights the importance of nurturing and supporting our gut health. By adopting lifestyle habits that promote a healthy gut, such as consuming a diverse and nutrient-rich diet, managing stress, getting regular physical activity, and avoiding harmful substances, we can optimize our gut health and enhance our overall well-being.

Gut Microbiota: Your Internal Ecosystem
Deep within your digestive system resides a vast and diverse community of microorganisms known as the gut

microbiota. This intricate ecosystem consists of trillions of bacteria, viruses, fungi, and other microscopic organisms that coexist in a delicate balance. While the idea of harboring so many microorganisms might seem unsettling, the truth is that these tiny inhabitants play a vital role in your overall health and well-being. In this chapter, we will explore the fascinating world of the gut microbiota and its significance for your internal ecosystem.

1. Diversity and Balance: A healthy gut microbiota thrives on diversity and balance. Just as a diverse ecosystem in nature is more resilient and sustainable, a diverse gut microbiota is associated with better health outcomes. The more diverse the microbial species in your gut, the better equipped it is to perform its various functions. Maintaining a balanced gut microbiota helps prevent the overgrowth of harmful bacteria and ensures that beneficial bacteria dominate the ecosystem.

2. Digestion and Nutrient Absorption: One of the primary roles of the gut microbiota is to aid in digestion and nutrient absorption. While our own digestive enzymes break down some components of our food, the gut microbiota helps to break down complex carbohydrates, fiber, and other indigestible compounds that our bodies can't process on their own. In return, they produce beneficial byproducts, such as short-chain fatty acids, that provide nourishment to the cells lining the gut.

3. Immune System Regulation: The gut microbiota plays a critical role in training and regulating our immune system. It interacts with immune cells and helps educate them to distinguish between harmful invaders and harmless substances. This interaction ensures that our immune system responds appropriately to threats while maintaining tolerance to beneficial microbes and food antigens. A well-balanced gut microbiota

supports a robust and well-regulated immune response.

4. Gut Barrier Function: The lining of the gut acts as a barrier, selectively allowing the absorption of nutrients while preventing harmful substances from entering the bloodstream. The gut microbiota helps maintain the integrity of this barrier by promoting the production of tight junction proteins and mucus, which create a physical barrier between the gut contents and the gut lining. This barrier function is crucial in preventing the leakage of toxins, undigested food particles, and harmful bacteria into the bloodstream.

5. Neurotransmitter Production: Surprisingly, the gut microbiota also contributes to the production of neurotransmitters, the chemical messengers that regulate communication between nerve cells. Some beneficial gut bacteria produce neurotransmitters such as serotonin,

dopamine, and GABA, which play essential roles in mood regulation, stress management, and cognitive function. The intricate gut-brain axis highlights the profound connection between the gut microbiota and mental well-being.

6. Metabolism and Weight Regulation: Emerging research suggests that the gut microbiota influences our metabolism and weight regulation. Certain microbes have been associated with a higher tendency to extract energy from food and store it as fat, potentially contributing to weight gain and obesity. Conversely, a diverse and balanced gut microbiota may support a more efficient metabolism and help maintain a healthy weight.

7. Communication with Other Organs: The gut microbiota communicates with other organs and systems in the body, exerting its influence beyond the digestive system. It can influence the function of the liver,

pancreas, and even the cardiovascular system. Imbalances in the gut microbiota have been linked to conditions such as fatty liver disease, insulin resistance, and cardiovascular disorders.

Understanding the significance of the gut microbiota as your internal ecosystem empowers you to take proactive steps in nurturing and supporting its health. By adopting a gut-friendly lifestyle, including a diverse and fiber-rich diet, regular exercise, stress management, and avoiding unnecessary antibiotic use, you can promote a healthy and balanced gut microbiota.

The Gut-Brain Axis: How Your Gut Influences Your Mood and Cognition

The connection between the gut and the brain is a complex and fascinating system known as the gut-brain axis. This bidirectional communication network involves constant interaction and signaling between the gut and the brain, shaping not only our digestive processes but also our mood, emotions, and cognitive function. Let's delve into the intricate relationship between the gut and the brain and explore how your gut influences your mood and cognition.

1. The Vagus Nerve: A major player in the gut-brain axis is the vagus nerve, which serves as a direct communication pathway between the gut and the brain. This nerve carries signals in both directions, allowing information to flow between the two systems. The gut microbiota produces neurotransmitters, such as serotonin, dopamine, and GABA, which travel along the vagus nerve and impact brain function and mood regulation.

2. Serotonin and Mood Regulation: Serotonin, often referred to as the "feel-good" neurotransmitter, plays a crucial role in regulating mood and emotions.

Interestingly, the majority of serotonin in our bodies is produced in the gut. The gut microbiota influences serotonin production and availability, directly impacting our mood. Imbalances in the gut microbiota have been associated with mood disorders, such as anxiety and depression.

3. Gut Hormones and Brain Function: The gut produces a variety of hormones that can influence brain function and cognition. For example, ghrelin, known as the hunger hormone, not only regulates appetite but also plays a role in memory and learning. Leptin, another gut hormone, is involved in the regulation of energy balance and can impact cognitive function. By modulating these gut hormones, the gut microbiota can indirectly affect brain health.

4. Inflammation and Brain Health: The gut-brain axis is closely intertwined with the immune system, and inflammation plays a pivotal role in this connection. Chronic

inflammation in the gut can lead to increased permeability of the gut lining, allowing harmful substances to enter the bloodstream. This can trigger systemic inflammation and activate the immune response in the brain, contributing to cognitive dysfunction and mood disorders.

5. Stress and Gut Health: The gut-brain axis is particularly sensitive to stress. Stress can disrupt the balance of the gut microbiota, increase gut permeability, and trigger inflammation in the gut. These effects can negatively impact brain function, mood, and cognition. Conversely, a healthy gut microbiota can help regulate the stress response and promote resilience to stress.

6. Microbial Metabolites and Brain Function: The gut microbiota produces a range of metabolites, such as short-chain fatty acids (SCFAs), that can influence brain function. SCFAs, like butyrate, have anti-inflammatory properties and can support the health of brain cells. They can

also enhance the production of neurotransmitters and promote neuroplasticity, the brain's ability to adapt and learn.

7. Probiotics and Mental Health: Probiotics, beneficial bacteria that can be consumed through certain foods or supplements, have shown promise in improving mental health outcomes. Some strains of probiotics have been associated with reduced symptoms of anxiety, depression, and stress. These beneficial bacteria can modulate the gut-brain axis, promote a healthy gut environment, and enhance mood and cognition.

Understanding the intricate relationship between the gut and the brain emphasizes the importance of nurturing a healthy gut for optimal mental well-being. By adopting habits that support gut health, such as consuming a diverse and fiber-rich diet, managing stress, getting regular exercise, and incorporating probiotic-rich foods, you can positively influence your mood and cognitive function. Let us now explore practical strategies to optimize your gut-brain axis and enhance your overall mental well-being.

Chapter 2: Signs and Symptoms of an Unhealthy Gut

Common gut-related issues and their symptoms

Our gut health plays a vital role in our overall well-being. When our gut is out of balance, it can manifest in a variety of signs and symptoms that may affect our daily lives. By recognizing these indicators, we can take proactive steps to restore our gut health and improve our overall wellness.

1. Digestive Issues: One of the primary indicators of an unhealthy gut is digestive discomfort. This may include symptoms such as bloating, gas, abdominal pain, constipation, diarrhea, or irregular bowel movements. These issues may stem from imbalances in gut bacteria, impaired digestion, or inflammation within the gastrointestinal tract.

2. Food Intolerances: If you find yourself experiencing adverse reactions to certain foods, it could be a sign of an unhealthy gut. Food intolerances, such as lactose or gluten intolerance, can develop when the gut lining becomes compromised, allowing undigested food particles to enter the bloodstream and trigger an immune response.

3. Fatigue and Low Energy: The gut has a significant impact on our energy levels. When our gut is not functioning optimally, nutrient absorption may be compromised, leading to nutrient deficiencies. This can result in fatigue, low energy levels, and a general sense of lethargy.

4. Mood Disorders: The gut and brain are intricately connected through the gut-brain axis. Research has shown that an unhealthy gut can contribute to mood disorders such as anxiety and depression. This is because the gut produces neurotransmitters like serotonin, which plays a crucial role in

regulating mood. Imbalances in gut bacteria can disrupt the production of these neurotransmitters, affecting our emotional well-being.

5. Skin Conditions: The health of our gut can also be reflected in our skin. Conditions such as acne, eczema, psoriasis, or rosacea may be indicative of an imbalanced gut. Inflammation and toxins produced by gut bacteria can contribute to skin inflammation and aggravate existing skin conditions.

6. Weakened Immune System: A significant portion of our immune system resides in the gut. When the gut is unhealthy, it can compromise the immune response, making us more susceptible to infections, frequent colds, and allergies. Recurring illnesses or a weakened immune system may signal an imbalance in gut health.

7. Brain Fog and Cognitive Issues: The gut-brain connection also affects cognitive function. Poor gut health has been linked to brain fog, difficulty concentrating, memory problems, and a decline in cognitive performance. The gut produces neurotransmitters and communicates with the brain through various pathways, influencing cognitive processes.

8. Weight Fluctuations: An unhealthy gut can contribute to weight imbalances. Some individuals may experience unexplained weight gain, while others may struggle with difficulty losing weight. Gut bacteria imbalances can affect the way our bodies extract and store energy from food, potentially leading to weight fluctuations.

It's important to remember that these signs and symptoms can vary from person to person, and it's always recommended to consult with a healthcare professional for a proper diagnosis. However, if you identify with several of these indicators, it may be a sign that your gut health needs attention.

Recognizing the Impact of an Imbalanced Gut on Your Well-being

Our gut health is intricately linked to our overall well-being. When our gut is imbalanced, it can have a profound impact on various aspects of our physical, mental, and emotional health. By understanding the far-reaching consequences of an imbalanced gut, we can become more attuned to the importance of nurturing and restoring our gut health.

1. Digestive Discomfort: Perhaps the most obvious impact of an imbalanced gut is digestive discomfort. You may experience symptoms such as bloating, gas, indigestion, diarrhea, or constipation. These issues arise from disruptions in the gut microbiota, inflammation in the digestive tract, or impaired digestive function. When our gut is out of balance, it struggles to

efficiently break down and absorb nutrients, leading to digestive distress.

2. Weakened Immune System: A healthy gut is crucial for a robust immune system. Approximately 70% of our immune system resides in the gut, and the gut microbiota plays a significant role in immune function. When the gut is imbalanced, with an overgrowth of harmful bacteria or a lack of beneficial bacteria, our immune system can become compromised. This can result in increased susceptibility to infections, allergies, and autoimmune disorders.

3. Inflammation and Chronic Conditions: Imbalances in the gut can contribute to chronic inflammation, which is linked to a wide range of health conditions. Inflammation in the gut can trigger a systemic inflammatory response throughout the body, leading to conditions such as inflammatory bowel disease (IBD), rheumatoid arthritis, asthma, and even

cardiovascular disease. Addressing gut health imbalances is crucial for managing and preventing chronic inflammation.

4. Mental and Emotional Well-being: The gut-brain axis, the communication network between the gut and the brain, highlights the strong connection between gut health and mental and emotional well-being. An imbalanced gut can disrupt the production and regulation of neurotransmitters, such as serotonin and dopamine, which play vital roles in mood regulation. This can contribute to symptoms of anxiety, depression, mood swings, and even cognitive decline.

5. Nutrient Deficiencies: When our gut is imbalanced, it can impair the absorption of essential nutrients from the foods we consume. Even if you have a healthy diet, an imbalanced gut may prevent proper absorption of key vitamins, minerals, and antioxidants. Over time, this can lead to

nutrient deficiencies, affecting various bodily functions and overall vitality.

6. Skin Conditions: The gut-skin connection highlights the impact of gut health on the health of our skin. An imbalanced gut can contribute to skin issues such as acne, eczema, psoriasis, and rosacea. Inflammation in the gut can trigger systemic inflammation, leading to skin inflammation and exacerbating existing skin conditions.

7. Energy and Fatigue: Our gut plays a crucial role in energy production. When our gut is imbalanced, nutrient absorption is compromised, leading to potential nutrient deficiencies. These deficiencies can result in low energy levels, chronic fatigue, and a general sense of lethargy.

By recognizing the impact of an imbalanced gut on your well-being, you can take proactive steps to restore balance and nurture your gut health.

Identifying the Root Causes of Gut Health Disturbances

Achieving optimal gut health requires identifying and addressing the root causes of gut disturbances. While each person's experience is unique, several common factors can contribute to imbalances in the gut microbiota and overall gut health. By understanding these root causes, you can make targeted changes to support your gut and promote long-term well-being.

1. Poor Diet: One of the primary culprits behind gut health disturbances is a poor diet. Consuming a diet high in processed foods, refined sugars, unhealthy fats, and low in fiber can negatively impact the gut microbiota. These dietary choices can promote the growth of harmful bacteria while suppressing the growth of beneficial bacteria. Over time, this imbalance can lead to inflammation, digestive issues, and compromised gut function.

2. Chronic Stress: Stress has a profound impact on our gut health. When we experience chronic stress, our body enters a state of heightened inflammation, which can disrupt the balance of the gut microbiota. Additionally, stress can affect gut motility, digestion, and nutrient absorption. Managing stress through practices such as meditation, deep breathing, and engaging in activities that promote relaxation is crucial for maintaining a healthy gut.

3. Antibiotics and Medications: While antibiotics are necessary to treat certain infections, they can disrupt the delicate balance of the gut microbiota. Antibiotics not only kill harmful bacteria but can also deplete beneficial bacteria, leading to gut dysbiosis. Additionally, other medications such as nonsteroidal anti-inflammatory drugs (NSAIDs) and proton pump inhibitors (PPIs) can also impact gut health. Whenever possible, it is important to work with healthcare professionals to minimize

the use of medications that may disrupt gut balance and explore alternative approaches when appropriate.

4. Environmental Factors: Environmental factors can also contribute to gut disturbances. Exposure to pollutants, toxins, and certain chemicals in our environment can have a detrimental effect on gut health. For example, pesticides found in conventionally grown foods can disrupt the gut microbiota. Additionally, exposure to environmental toxins such as heavy metals can negatively impact gut function. Choosing organic foods when possible and minimizing exposure to harmful environmental factors can support a healthy gut.

5. Lack of Physical Activity: Sedentary lifestyles can contribute to gut health imbalances. Regular physical activity promotes gut motility, which aids in efficient digestion and elimination. Exercise also

helps to reduce stress levels, support a healthy immune response, and promote overall well-being. Incorporating movement into your daily routine, whether through structured exercise or active hobbies, can positively influence your gut health.

6. Insufficient Sleep: Sleep plays a vital role in maintaining overall health, including gut health. Inadequate sleep or poor sleep quality can disrupt the delicate balance of the gut microbiota and impair gut function. Aim for consistent, quality sleep by establishing a relaxing bedtime routine, creating a conducive sleep environment, and prioritizing restful sleep.

7. Food Sensitivities and Allergies: Undiagnosed food sensitivities or allergies can contribute to gut disturbances. Certain foods, such as gluten, dairy, or specific types of carbohydrates, may trigger inflammation or adverse reactions in the gut. Identifying and eliminating foods that cause

sensitivities can help restore gut balance and alleviate symptoms.

By identifying and addressing these root causes, you can take proactive steps to restore gut health and support your overall well-being.

Chapter 3: Nurturing Your Gut: A Holistic Approach

The Importance of a Balanced and Diverse Diet for Gut Health

When it comes to maintaining a healthy gut, one of the most crucial factors is a balanced and diverse diet. The foods we eat directly impact the composition and function of our gut microbiota, which in turn affects our overall gut health. In this section, we will explore the importance of a balanced and diverse diet for promoting optimal gut health.

1. Providing Essential Nutrients: A balanced diet ensures that your body receives all the necessary nutrients it needs to function properly. This includes essential vitamins, minerals, fiber, and antioxidants that support various aspects of gut health. Fiber, in particular, is important for promoting a healthy gut. It acts as a prebiotic, serving as

a fuel source for beneficial gut bacteria and helping them thrive.

2. Supporting Microbial Diversity: The gut microbiota is composed of trillions of microorganisms, including bacteria, fungi, and viruses. Having a diverse range of gut bacteria is associated with better overall health. A balanced diet rich in a variety of fruits, vegetables, whole grains, legumes, and fermented foods can help foster microbial diversity in the gut. Each type of food introduces different beneficial compounds and nutrients that support the growth of diverse bacterial species.

3. Promoting Gut Barrier Function: The gut lining acts as a barrier between the contents of the gut and the bloodstream. A healthy gut barrier is essential for preventing the entry of harmful substances and pathogens into the body. Certain foods, such as those rich in omega-3 fatty acids, antioxidants, and polyphenols, can help strengthen the

gut barrier, reducing inflammation and maintaining its integrity.

4. Enhancing Digestion and Absorption: A balanced diet supports optimal digestion and nutrient absorption. It provides an adequate amount of dietary fiber, which adds bulk to the stool and promotes regular bowel movements. This helps prevent constipation and supports the elimination of waste products from the body. Additionally, a diverse range of gut bacteria helps break down complex carbohydrates and fiber, aiding in the absorption of nutrients from the food we consume.

5. Reducing Inflammation: Chronic inflammation in the gut can disrupt the balance of the gut microbiota and lead to various gut health issues. A diet rich in processed foods, refined sugars, unhealthy fats, and artificial additives can promote inflammation in the body. On the other hand, a balanced diet that focuses on whole,

unprocessed foods can help reduce inflammation and support a healthier gut environment.

6. Modulating Gut Hormones: Certain foods can influence the release of gut hormones, which play a role in appetite regulation, metabolism, and digestion. For example, foods high in fiber can promote feelings of fullness and help maintain a healthy weight. Consuming a balanced diet that includes a variety of nutrients and food groups can help keep gut hormones in balance, supporting overall gut health.

To optimize your gut health through diet, aim for a varied and balanced eating pattern. Include a wide range of fruits, vegetables, whole grains, legumes, nuts, seeds, lean proteins, and fermented foods in your meals. Experiment with different flavors, textures, and cooking methods to make your meals enjoyable and diverse. Remember to stay hydrated and listen to your body's cues of hunger and fullness.

By prioritizing a balanced and diverse diet, you can nourish your gut microbiota, support gut barrier function, reduce inflammation, and promote optimal digestion and nutrient absorption. Take this opportunity to explore new recipes, try different cuisines, and discover the joy of nourishing your gut and overall well-being through the power of food.

Nutritional Strategies for Promoting Gut Health

Taking care of your gut health goes beyond just eating a balanced and diverse diet. It also involves implementing specific nutritional strategies that can further support the well-being of your gut. In this section, we will explore some key nutritional strategies you can incorporate into your daily routine to promote optimal gut health.

1. Consume Prebiotic Foods: Prebiotics are a type of fiber that serve as food for the beneficial bacteria in your gut. Including prebiotic-rich foods in your diet can help nourish and support the growth of these beneficial bacteria. Some examples of prebiotic foods include onions, garlic, leeks, asparagus, bananas, oats, and flaxseeds. Aim to incorporate these foods into your meals regularly to enhance your gut microbiota.

2. Include Probiotic-Rich Foods: Probiotics are live beneficial bacteria that can directly introduce new strains of bacteria into your gut. Consuming foods that are naturally rich in probiotics can help replenish and diversify your gut microbiota. Some common probiotic-rich foods include yogurt, kefir, sauerkraut, kimchi, miso, and kombucha. Consider adding these foods to your diet to introduce beneficial bacteria and promote a healthy gut environment.

3. Consider Probiotic Supplements: In addition to consuming probiotic-rich foods, you may also consider incorporating probiotic supplements into your routine. These supplements contain specific strains of beneficial bacteria in concentrated form, offering a convenient way to boost your gut microbiota. When choosing a probiotic supplement, look for a reputable brand that offers a variety of strains and a high number of colony-forming units (CFUs).

4. Focus on Anti-Inflammatory Foods: Chronic inflammation in the gut can disrupt the balance of the gut microbiota and contribute to gut health issues. Including anti-inflammatory foods in your diet can help reduce inflammation and support a healthier gut environment. Such foods include fatty fish rich in omega-3 fatty acids, leafy greens, berries, turmeric, ginger, olive oil, and walnuts. Incorporate these foods into your meals to provide your gut with anti-inflammatory compounds.

5. Emphasize Fiber-Rich Foods: Dietary fiber plays a crucial role in maintaining a healthy gut. It provides fuel for the beneficial bacteria in your gut, promotes regular bowel movements, and helps prevent constipation. Include a variety of fiber-rich foods in your diet, such as whole grains, fruits, vegetables, legumes, and nuts. Aim for the recommended daily intake of fiber, which is around 25-38 grams for adults, depending on age and gender.

6. Stay Hydrated: Drinking an adequate amount of water is essential for maintaining a healthy gut. Water helps soften the stool, making it easier to pass and preventing constipation. It also supports the proper digestion and absorption of nutrients. Aim to drink enough water throughout the day to stay hydrated and support your gut health.

7. Practice Mindful Eating: Mindful eating involves paying attention to the sensory

experience of eating, including the taste, texture, and aroma of food. It also involves listening to your body's hunger and fullness cues. By practicing mindful eating, you can promote proper digestion, enhance nutrient absorption, and avoid overeating. Take the time to savor and enjoy your meals, and try to minimize distractions while eating.

By incorporating these nutritional strategies into your daily routine, you can take proactive steps to support your gut health. Remember that everyone's gut is unique, so it's important to listen to your body and find the dietary approach that works best for you. Experiment with different foods, flavors, and cooking methods to discover what nourishes your gut and promotes optimal well-being.

Gut-Friendly Foods and Their Benefits

When it comes to promoting gut health, certain foods have been shown to have particularly beneficial effects on the gut microbiota and overall digestive well-being. Including these gut-friendly foods in your diet can provide a range of nutrients and compounds that support a healthy gut environment. Let's explore some of these foods and their specific benefits:

1. Yogurt: Yogurt is a well-known source of probiotics, which are beneficial bacteria that can help restore and maintain a healthy gut microbiota. Probiotics in yogurt, such as Lactobacillus and Bifidobacterium strains, promote gut balance and support digestion. Additionally, yogurt is a good source of calcium and protein, which contribute to overall bone health and muscle maintenance.

2. Kefir: Similar to yogurt, kefir is a fermented dairy product that contains a variety of probiotic strains. It is rich in beneficial bacteria and yeasts, providing a diverse range of microorganisms for your gut. Kefir is also a good source of vitamins,

minerals, and amino acids, making it a nutritious addition to your diet.

3. Sauerkraut: Sauerkraut is a fermented cabbage dish that is rich in probiotics and enzymes. The fermentation process enhances the bioavailability of nutrients in cabbage and promotes the growth of beneficial bacteria. Consuming sauerkraut can support digestion, improve nutrient absorption, and boost immune function.

4. Kimchi: Kimchi is a traditional Korean dish made from fermented vegetables, primarily cabbage and radishes. It is packed with probiotics, vitamins, and minerals. Kimchi is known for its spicy and tangy flavor and is a versatile addition to various meals. Regular consumption of kimchi can contribute to a healthy gut microbiota and overall digestive health.

5. Kombucha: Kombucha is a fermented tea beverage that is naturally carbonated. It is

made by fermenting sweetened tea with a symbiotic culture of bacteria and yeast (SCOBY). Kombucha contains probiotics, organic acids, and antioxidants that support gut health. It has gained popularity for its potential benefits in improving digestion, immune function, and overall well-being.

6. Whole Grains: Whole grains, such as oats, quinoa, brown rice, and whole wheat, are excellent sources of dietary fiber. Fiber acts as a prebiotic, nourishing the beneficial bacteria in your gut and promoting their growth. Whole grains also provide essential nutrients like B vitamins and minerals. Including whole grains in your diet can support regular bowel movements and contribute to a healthy gut environment.

7. Fruits and Vegetables: A wide variety of fruits and vegetables are beneficial for gut health due to their high fiber content, as well as their vitamins, minerals, and antioxidants. Examples of gut-friendly fruits include

berries, apples, bananas, and citrus fruits. Leafy green vegetables, cruciferous vegetables (such as broccoli and kale), and root vegetables (such as carrots and sweet potatoes) are also beneficial. These foods provide essential nutrients and support a healthy gut microbiota.

8. Ginger: Ginger has long been used for its medicinal properties, including its ability to aid digestion and alleviate gastrointestinal discomfort. It has anti-inflammatory and antioxidant properties that can support gut health. Ginger can be enjoyed in various forms, such as fresh ginger root, ginger tea, or added to dishes and smoothies.

9. Turmeric: Turmeric contains a compound called curcumin, which has anti-inflammatory and antioxidant properties. It can help reduce inflammation in the gut and support overall digestive health. Turmeric is commonly used in

curries, golden milk, and various other dishes.

10. Bone Broth: Bone broth is made by simmering bones and connective tissues, such as chicken or beef bones

, for an extended period. It is rich in nutrients like collagen, gelatin, and amino acids, which can support gut healing and repair. Bone broth is a soothing and nourishing beverage that can be enjoyed on its own or used as a base for soups and stews.

Incorporating these gut-friendly foods into your diet can provide a range of benefits, including supporting a diverse and balanced gut microbiota, promoting digestion, reducing inflammation, and enhancing nutrient absorption. Remember to choose high-quality, organic, and minimally processed versions of these foods whenever possible to maximize their nutritional value.

Gut-Healing Herbs and Supplements

In addition to incorporating gut-friendly foods into your diet, certain herbs and supplements can provide additional support for gut healing and overall digestive well-being. These natural remedies can help reduce inflammation, support the growth of beneficial gut bacteria, and promote a healthy gut environment. Let's explore some gut-healing herbs and supplements that you may consider incorporating into your routine:

1. Aloe Vera: Aloe vera has long been recognized for its soothing properties and its ability to support digestive health. It can help soothe inflamed tissues in the gut and promote healing. Aloe vera gel or juice can be consumed internally to support gut health and relieve gastrointestinal discomfort.

2. Slippery Elm: Slippery elm is an herb known for its mucilage content, which forms a gel-like substance when mixed with water. This gel can coat and soothe the lining of the gastrointestinal tract, reducing inflammation and promoting healing. Slippery elm can be consumed as a tea or in supplement form.

3. Marshmallow Root: Marshmallow root also contains mucilage, which can provide a protective and soothing effect on the gut lining. It can help relieve symptoms of digestive issues, such as irritation, inflammation, and discomfort. Marshmallow root can be consumed as a tea, in capsule form, or as a powder.

4. Probiotic Supplements: Probiotic supplements are concentrated forms of beneficial bacteria that can help restore and maintain a healthy gut microbiota. They can be especially beneficial if you have experienced gut imbalances or if your diet

lacks probiotic-rich foods. Look for a high-quality probiotic supplement that contains a variety of strains and a high number of colony-forming units (CFUs).

5. Digestive Enzymes: Digestive enzymes are naturally occurring substances in our bodies that help break down food and facilitate proper digestion. However, certain factors like age, diet, and gut health issues can affect the production and effectiveness of these enzymes. Taking digestive enzyme supplements can aid in the digestion and absorption of nutrients, relieving digestive discomfort and supporting gut health.

6. L-Glutamine: L-Glutamine is an amino acid that plays a vital role in maintaining the integrity and function of the gut lining. It supports the growth and repair of intestinal cells and helps reduce inflammation in the gut. L-Glutamine supplements can be beneficial for individuals with gut health

issues, such as leaky gut syndrome or gastrointestinal inflammation.

7. Omega-3 Fatty Acids: Omega-3 fatty acids, found in fatty fish like salmon, mackerel, and sardines, have anti-inflammatory properties that can support gut health. If your diet is lacking in omega-3 fatty acids, you may consider taking fish oil supplements to provide these essential nutrients and promote a healthy inflammatory response in the gut.

8. Curcumin: Curcumin, the active compound in turmeric, has powerful anti-inflammatory and antioxidant properties. It can help reduce inflammation in the gut and support overall digestive health. Curcumin supplements can be beneficial for individuals with gut-related inflammation or inflammatory bowel diseases.

9. Zinc: Zinc is a mineral that plays a crucial role in maintaining a healthy gut lining. It supports the integrity of the intestinal barrier and helps promote healing and repair. Zinc supplements can be beneficial for individuals with gut health issues or zinc deficiencies.

10. Fiber Supplements: If your diet lacks sufficient fiber, you may consider adding fiber supplements to support gut health. These supplements can provide additional fiber to nourish the beneficial bacteria in your gut and promote regular bowel movements. Look for soluble fiber supplements, such as psyllium husk or acacia fiber, that can easily be added to your diet.

Remember to consult with a healthcare professional or a registered dietitian before starting any new supplements, as they can provide personalized guidance based on your specific health needs and considerations.

Chapter 4: The Gut-Brain Connection: Boosting Mental and Emotional Wellness

Exploring the Link Between Gut Health and Mental Health

In recent years, there has been growing evidence to suggest a strong connection between gut health and mental health. The gut-brain axis, a bidirectional communication network between the gut and the brain, plays a crucial role in this relationship. Emerging research has highlighted the influence of gut microbiota on various aspects of mental well-being, including mood, cognition, and even certain mental health disorders. Let's delve deeper into the fascinating link between gut health and mental health:

1. Gut Microbiota and Neurotransmitters: The gut microbiota, the trillions of

microorganisms residing in your gut, have a significant impact on the production and regulation of neurotransmitters, the chemical messengers in the brain that influence mood and cognition. For example, certain beneficial gut bacteria produce neurotransmitters like serotonin, which is commonly known as the "feel-good" hormone. An imbalance in gut microbiota can affect neurotransmitter levels, potentially contributing to mood disorders such as depression and anxiety.

2. Inflammation and Mental Health: Chronic inflammation in the body, including in the gut, has been linked to various mental health conditions. Imbalances in the gut microbiota can lead to increased intestinal permeability (leaky gut), allowing harmful substances to enter the bloodstream and trigger an inflammatory response. This chronic low-grade inflammation can negatively impact brain function and contribute to mental health disorders.

3. Communication via the Vagus Nerve: The gut and the brain communicate through the vagus nerve, which serves as a major pathway for information exchange between the two. Signals from the gut can influence brain function, emotions, and behavior. This bidirectional communication suggests that changes in gut health can have a profound impact on mental well-being.

4. The Role of Short-Chain Fatty Acids (SCFAs): The gut microbiota produce short-chain fatty acids (SCFAs) as a byproduct of fermenting dietary fiber. SCFAs, such as butyrate, acetate, and propionate, have been shown to have anti-inflammatory properties and provide energy for the cells lining the gut. They also play a role in regulating the immune system and influencing brain function. Imbalances in SCFAs have been associated with mental health conditions, emphasizing the

importance of a healthy gut microbiota and adequate dietary fiber intake.

5. Stress Response and Gut Health: Stress, whether acute or chronic, can have a significant impact on gut health. Stress activates the release of stress hormones, which can alter the composition of the gut microbiota and increase intestinal permeability. This disruption in gut health can further perpetuate stress-related symptoms and impact mental well-being. Nurturing a healthy gut can help support a resilient stress response.

6. Gut Health Interventions for Mental Health: Several studies have explored the potential therapeutic effects of interventions targeting gut health for mental health conditions. Probiotics, which are beneficial bacteria, have shown promise in improving symptoms of depression, anxiety, and stress. Prebiotics, which serve as food for beneficial gut bacteria, can also support a

healthy gut microbiota and potentially have positive effects on mental health. Additionally, dietary and lifestyle modifications that promote gut health, such as a nutrient-dense diet, regular exercise, stress management techniques, and adequate sleep, can contribute to overall mental well-being.

Understanding the intricate relationship between gut health and mental health opens up new avenues for holistic approaches to mental well-being. Taking care of your gut through a balanced diet, stress management, and targeted interventions can have a positive impact on your mental health and overall quality of life. It is important to consult with a healthcare professional for personalized guidance and to explore appropriate strategies that suit your individual needs.

Strategies for Reducing Stress and Promoting Relaxation

In our fast-paced and demanding lives, stress has become a common companion. Chronic stress not only takes a toll on our mental well-being but also impacts our physical health. It is crucial to find effective strategies to reduce stress and promote relaxation. Here are some strategies that can help you unwind, find inner calm, and restore balance in your life:

1. Practice Mindfulness: Mindfulness is the practice of being fully present and aware of the present moment without judgment. Engaging in mindfulness exercises, such as meditation or deep breathing, can help calm your mind, reduce anxiety, and improve your overall sense of well-being. Dedicate a few minutes each day to sit in a quiet space, focus on your breath, and observe your thoughts without getting caught up in them.

2. Engage in Physical Activity: Physical activity is not only beneficial for your physical health but also for your mental well-being. Engaging in regular exercise, whether it's a brisk walk, yoga, dancing, or any form of movement that you enjoy, releases endorphins, the "feel-good" hormones, and helps reduce stress. Find activities that you genuinely enjoy and incorporate them into your daily routine.

3. Connect with Nature: Spending time in nature has a soothing and calming effect on the mind and body. Take a walk in a park, hike in the mountains, or simply sit in your backyard and observe the beauty of the natural world. Disconnect from technology and immerse yourself in the sights, sounds, and scents of nature. It can help reduce stress, improve your mood, and provide a sense of peace and tranquility.

4. Practice Relaxation Techniques: Explore various relaxation techniques to find what

works best for you. Deep breathing exercises, progressive muscle relaxation, guided imagery, or listening to calming music can all help induce a state of relaxation. Dedicate a specific time each day to engage in these techniques, especially during moments of heightened stress or when you need a break from the daily hustle and bustle.

5. Cultivate Healthy Coping Mechanisms: Everyone has different ways of coping with stress, but it's important to develop healthy coping mechanisms that promote relaxation rather than exacerbating stress. Engage in activities that bring you joy and help you unwind, such as reading, listening to music, taking a warm bath, practicing hobbies, or spending quality time with loved ones. Find what resonates with you and prioritize self-care activities that nourish your mind, body, and soul.

6. Prioritize Sleep: Sleep is a fundamental pillar of well-being, and quality sleep plays a vital role in stress management. Establish a consistent sleep routine, create a sleep-friendly environment, and practice relaxation techniques before bed to promote restful sleep. Prioritize adequate sleep duration to rejuvenate your mind and body and wake up feeling refreshed and ready to face the day.

7. Seek Support: Don't hesitate to reach out for support when needed. Talk to trusted friends or family members about your stressors and feelings. Consider seeking professional help from a therapist or counselor who can provide guidance and support in managing stress. Surround yourself with a supportive network of individuals who understand and validate your experiences.

Remember, finding effective strategies for reducing stress and promoting relaxation is a personal journey. Experiment with different techniques, be patient with yourself, and find a combination of strategies that work best for you. By incorporating these practices into your daily life, you can create a healthier relationship with stress, cultivate inner peace, and enhance your overall well-being.

Mindful Eating for Gut and Brain Harmony

In our fast-paced and busy lives, we often find ourselves rushing through meals, eating on the go, or mindlessly consuming food without paying attention to the experience. However, practicing mindful eating can have profound benefits for both our gut and brain health. It involves bringing awareness and intention to the act of eating, savoring each bite, and cultivating a deeper connection with our body's needs. Here's how mindful eating can promote gut and brain harmony:

1. Enhances Digestion: Mindful eating allows us to slow down and fully engage with our meal. By paying attention to the colors, smells, textures, and flavors of the food, we activate our senses and enhance the digestive process. Chewing food thoroughly and savoring each bite helps break down food more effectively, leading to improved digestion and nutrient absorption.

2. Supports Healthy Eating Habits: Mindful eating encourages a more conscious and intentional approach to food choices. By tuning into our body's hunger and fullness cues, we can make choices that align with our nutritional needs rather than emotional or external triggers. This can help prevent overeating, support portion control, and promote a balanced and nourishing diet.

3. Promotes Gut-Brain Connection: The gut and brain are intricately connected through the gut-brain axis, a complex network of communication pathways. Mindful eating

can positively influence this connection. When we eat mindfully, we reduce stress and activate the parasympathetic nervous system, which is responsible for rest and digestion. This can enhance gut health, reduce digestive discomfort, and positively impact our mood and mental well-being.

4. Heightens Food Appreciation: Mindful eating invites us to fully appreciate the taste, aroma, and texture of our food. By taking the time to savor each bite, we develop a deeper connection with the nourishment that food provides. This heightened appreciation can lead to a greater sense of satisfaction and enjoyment from our meals, which in turn supports our overall well-being.

5. Reduces Emotional Eating: Many of us turn to food as a source of comfort or distraction during times of stress or emotional turmoil. Mindful eating helps us become more aware of our emotional triggers and develop a greater

understanding of our relationship with food. By practicing non-judgmental awareness, we can cultivate healthier coping mechanisms and break free from emotional eating patterns.

6. Cultivates Mind-Body Awareness: Mindful eating is an opportunity to connect with our body and listen to its needs. It helps us tune into sensations of hunger, fullness, and satisfaction. By cultivating this mind-body awareness, we can make conscious choices that honor our physical and emotional well-being. This awareness extends beyond mealtime and can positively impact our overall lifestyle choices.

Incorporating Mindful Eating into Your Routine:
1. Slow down: Take your time while eating, and savor each bite. Put down your utensils between bites and engage your senses in the eating experience.

2. Engage your senses: Notice the colors, smells, and textures of your food. Take a moment to appreciate the flavors and the nourishment they provide.

3. Practice gratitude: Before each meal, express gratitude for the food on your plate and the efforts that went into its production. This practice can foster a sense of appreciation and mindfulness.

4. Listen to your body: Pay attention to your body's hunger and fullness cues. Eat when you are truly hungry and stop when you feel comfortably satisfied.

5. Minimize distractions: Create a calm and peaceful eating environment by minimizing distractions like screens or multitasking. Focus solely on the act of eating and being present in the moment.

6. Practice self-compassion: Be gentle with yourself throughout the process. Let go of

judgment or guilt surrounding food choices and embrace a compassionate attitude towards yourself and your body.

By incorporating mindful eating into your daily routine, you can cultivate a harmonious relationship between your gut and brain. It not only enhances your digestion and nutrient absorption but also supports healthy eating habits, reduces emotional eating, and promotes overall well-being. Embrace the practice of mindful eating as a powerful tool for nourishing both your body and mind.

Gut-Nourishing Practices for Emotional Well-Being

Our gut health and emotional well-being are deeply interconnected. The state of our gut can influence our mood, stress levels, and overall emotional balance. By adopting gut-nourishing practices, we can support both our physical and emotional health. Here are some practices to incorporate into your daily routine to nourish your gut and promote emotional well-being:

1. Eat a Balanced and Fiber-Rich Diet: A diet that is rich in fiber helps promote a healthy gut microbiota. Include a variety of fruits, vegetables, whole grains, legumes, and nuts in your meals to provide your gut with the essential nutrients and dietary fiber it needs. These fiber-rich foods also help regulate blood sugar levels, support stable energy levels, and contribute to a positive mood.

2. Prioritize Probiotic Foods: Probiotics are beneficial bacteria that can promote a healthy gut microbiome. Incorporate fermented foods like yogurt, sauerkraut, kimchi, kefir, and tempeh into your diet. These foods help introduce beneficial bacteria into your gut, which can enhance digestion, boost nutrient absorption, and support a balanced mood.

3. Stay Hydrated: Drinking an adequate amount of water is essential for maintaining proper digestion and gut health. Water helps transport nutrients, aids in waste elimination, and ensures the smooth functioning of the digestive system. Aim to drink at least 8 glasses of water per day to stay hydrated and support optimal gut function.

4. Manage Stress: Chronic stress can negatively impact both your gut and emotional well-being. Practice stress management techniques such as meditation, deep breathing exercises, yoga, or mindfulness to help reduce stress levels. Engaging in activities that bring you joy, like spending time in nature, practicing hobbies, or connecting with loved ones, can also help alleviate stress and promote emotional balance.

5. Get Regular Exercise: Regular physical activity not only supports overall health but

also benefits gut health and emotional well-being. Exercise helps stimulate bowel movements, improves digestion, and promotes the release of endorphins, which are natural mood enhancers. Find activities you enjoy, such as walking, jogging, dancing, or cycling, and aim for at least 30 minutes of exercise most days of the week.

6. Prioritize Sleep: Quality sleep is crucial for both gut health and emotional well-being. Aim to get 7-9 hours of uninterrupted sleep each night to allow your body and mind to rest and rejuvenate. Establish a relaxing bedtime routine, create a comfortable sleep environment, and limit exposure to electronic devices before bed to promote better sleep quality.

7. Practice Mindful Eating: Mindful eating, as discussed earlier, involves being fully present and attentive to the act of eating. When we eat mindfully, we are more likely to make nourishing food choices, chew our

food thoroughly, and support optimal digestion. Mindful eating can also help us develop a positive relationship with food and cultivate a sense of gratitude for the nourishment it provides.

8. Seek Emotional Support: It is important to recognize when you need emotional support and reach out to trusted friends, family members, or professionals. Sharing your thoughts and feelings with others can provide a sense of connection, understanding, and validation. Professional support from therapists or counselors can offer guidance and help navigate emotional challenges effectively.

Remember, nourishing your gut is not just about the food you eat but also the practices you incorporate into your daily life. By adopting these gut-nourishing practices, you can support your emotional well-being, cultivate a healthier gut environment, and foster a greater sense of balance and harmony in your life. Prioritize self-care, listen to your body's needs, and make choices that nourish your gut and nourish your soul.

Chapter 5: Healing Your Gut: Restoring Balance and Repairing Damage

Understanding Leaky Gut Syndrome and Its Implications

Leaky gut syndrome, also known as increased intestinal permeability, is a condition that has gained attention in recent years for its potential impact on overall health and well-being. It refers to a condition where the lining of the intestinal wall becomes compromised, allowing undigested food particles, toxins, and bacteria to leak into the bloodstream. This leakage triggers an immune response and can lead to a range of health issues. Here, we delve into understanding leaky gut syndrome and its implications:

1. The Gut Barrier: The lining of the intestines acts as a barrier, selectively allowing the absorption of nutrients while

preventing harmful substances from entering the bloodstream. This barrier is made up of tight junctions, which are protein structures that hold the intestinal cells together. When these junctions become damaged or weakened, gaps may form, resulting in the leaky gut condition.

2. Causes and Contributing Factors: Several factors can contribute to the development of leaky gut syndrome. These include poor diet choices, chronic stress, excessive alcohol consumption, prolonged use of non-steroidal anti-inflammatory drugs (NSAIDs), certain medications, intestinal infections, imbalanced gut microbiota, and environmental toxins. These factors can disrupt the delicate balance of the gut environment and compromise the integrity of the gut lining.

3. Implications for Health: Leaky gut syndrome has been linked to various health issues and may have implications beyond

the digestive system. When substances leak into the bloodstream, the immune system can mount an immune response, leading to inflammation throughout the body. Chronic inflammation is associated with conditions such as autoimmune diseases, allergies, skin problems, hormonal imbalances, mood disorders, and even neurological conditions. Additionally, the compromised gut barrier may hinder proper nutrient absorption, potentially leading to nutrient deficiencies and further health complications.

4. Symptoms and Signs: The symptoms of leaky gut syndrome can vary widely and may manifest differently in each individual. Common signs include bloating, gas, abdominal pain, diarrhea, constipation, fatigue, brain fog, skin rashes, joint pain, food sensitivities, and mood disturbances. However, it's important to note that these symptoms can overlap with other conditions, making it challenging to diagnose leaky gut solely based on symptoms.

5. Diagnosis and Treatment: Diagnosing leaky gut syndrome can be complex, as there is no single definitive test available. However, healthcare professionals may consider a combination of medical history, symptoms, laboratory tests, and elimination diets to assess the presence of leaky gut. Treatment typically involves addressing the underlying causes and supporting gut healing. This may include dietary modifications (such as eliminating inflammatory foods, promoting gut-friendly foods, and incorporating healing nutrients), managing stress levels, optimizing sleep, taking supplements that support gut health (such as probiotics, digestive enzymes, and L-glutamine), and working closely with healthcare professionals to develop a personalized treatment plan.

6. Lifestyle Considerations: Making lifestyle changes can significantly contribute to healing a leaky gut. Prioritizing a

nutrient-dense, whole-food diet rich in fiber, antioxidants, and anti-inflammatory foods can support gut healing. Managing stress through relaxation techniques, regular exercise, and adequate sleep can also play a vital role in supporting overall gut health. Additionally, avoiding or minimizing exposure to environmental toxins and adopting healthy lifestyle habits can further support the healing process.

Understanding leaky gut syndrome and its implications empowers individuals to take proactive steps towards gut health and overall well-being. While more research is needed to fully understand this complex condition, adopting a holistic approach that addresses the root causes and supports gut healing can promote a healthier gut environment and contribute to improved overall health. It is recommended to consult with a healthcare professional for proper diagnosis, guidance, and personalized treatment options.

Gut-Healing Protocols and Dietary Approaches

When it comes to healing the gut and addressing conditions like leaky gut syndrome, implementing specific protocols and dietary approaches can be beneficial. These protocols and approaches aim to reduce inflammation, support gut healing, restore balance to the gut microbiota, and promote overall digestive wellness. Here are some gut-healing protocols and dietary approaches to consider:

1. Elimination Diet: An elimination diet involves temporarily removing common inflammatory or allergenic foods from your diet. This approach helps identify potential food triggers that may be contributing to gut inflammation and exacerbating symptoms. Common foods to eliminate during the initial phase of an elimination diet include gluten, dairy, soy, corn, eggs, processed sugars, and artificial additives. After a period of elimination, these foods are gradually

reintroduced to observe any reactions or sensitivities.

2. Low-FODMAP Diet: The low-FODMAP diet is commonly used to manage symptoms of irritable bowel syndrome (IBS) and other gastrointestinal disorders. FODMAPs are fermentable carbohydrates that can be difficult to digest for some individuals, leading to symptoms such as bloating, gas, and abdominal pain. The low-FODMAP diet involves temporarily reducing or eliminating foods high in FODMAPs, such as certain fruits, vegetables, legumes, and grains. It is typically done under the guidance of a healthcare professional or registered dietitian.

3. Gut-Healing Nutrients: Certain nutrients play a crucial role in gut health and healing. Including foods rich in these nutrients can support the repair and regeneration of the gut lining. Examples of gut-healing nutrients

include L-glutamine, zinc, omega-3 fatty acids, vitamin A, vitamin D, and collagen. Incorporating foods such as bone broth, fatty fish, leafy greens, colorful vegetables, nuts, seeds, and fermented foods can provide these important nutrients.

4. Probiotics and Fermented Foods: Probiotics are beneficial bacteria that can help restore balance to the gut microbiota. Including probiotic-rich foods such as yogurt, kefir, sauerkraut, kimchi, and kombucha in your diet can introduce beneficial bacteria to support gut health. Additionally, fermented foods contain natural enzymes and beneficial bacteria that aid in digestion and promote a healthy gut environment.

5. Fiber-Rich Foods: Dietary fiber is essential for maintaining a healthy gut. It helps promote regular bowel movements, provides nourishment for the beneficial gut bacteria, and supports overall digestive

health. Include a variety of fiber-rich foods in your diet, such as fruits, vegetables, whole grains, legumes, and seeds.

6. Anti-Inflammatory Foods: Chronic inflammation in the gut can contribute to gut dysfunction and related symptoms. Including anti-inflammatory foods in your diet can help reduce inflammation and support gut healing. Some examples of anti-inflammatory foods include fatty fish (rich in omega-3 fatty acids), olive oil, turmeric, ginger, green leafy vegetables, berries, and nuts.

7. Adequate Hydration: Staying hydrated is crucial for optimal gut health. Drinking an adequate amount of water helps support digestion, nutrient absorption, and overall bowel regularity. Aim to drink at least 8 glasses of water per day and increase your intake if you are physically active or in hot weather.

Remember, it is essential to work with a healthcare professional or a registered dietitian to determine the most appropriate gut-healing protocol or dietary approach for your specific needs. They can provide personalized guidance, monitor your progress, and ensure that your nutritional needs are met throughout the healing process. Healing the gut takes time and patience, but by implementing these protocols and dietary approaches, you can support your gut health and pave the way for improved digestion and overall wellness.

Restoring Gut Health through Lifestyle Modifications

In addition to dietary changes, certain lifestyle modifications can significantly contribute to restoring gut health and promoting overall digestive wellness. These lifestyle factors can support the healing process, reduce inflammation, optimize digestion, and foster a healthy gut microbiota. Here are some key lifestyle modifications to consider:

1. Manage Stress: Chronic stress can have a detrimental impact on gut health. When you're under stress, the body's stress response can disrupt the delicate balance of the gut, leading to digestive issues and inflammation. Incorporate stress management techniques into your daily routine, such as mindfulness meditation, deep breathing exercises, yoga, or engaging in activities that bring you joy and relaxation. Finding healthy ways to cope with stress can help support a healthy gut environment.

2. Prioritize Sleep: Quality sleep is essential for overall health, including gut health. Lack of sleep or poor sleep quality can disrupt the gut-brain axis, leading to imbalances in gut bacteria and increased inflammation. Aim for 7-8 hours of uninterrupted sleep each

night and establish a regular sleep routine that promotes relaxation and restful sleep.

3. Exercise Regularly: Engaging in regular physical activity has numerous benefits for gut health. Exercise helps stimulate digestion, improves bowel regularity, and enhances blood flow to the intestines. It also contributes to overall stress reduction and supports a healthy immune system. Find activities you enjoy, whether it's walking, cycling, yoga, or dancing, and strive for at least 30 minutes of moderate-intensity exercise most days of the week.

4. Avoid Harmful Substances: Certain substances can disrupt the delicate balance of the gut and hinder gut healing. Minimize or avoid exposure to substances that can irritate the gut lining, such as tobacco, excessive alcohol, and non-steroidal anti-inflammatory drugs (NSAIDs) unless prescribed by a healthcare professional. Additionally, be mindful of environmental

toxins and pollutants that can contribute to gut inflammation. Opt for natural, non-toxic cleaning and personal care products to reduce your exposure.

5. Stay Hydrated: Drinking an adequate amount of water is crucial for maintaining a healthy gut. Water helps support digestion, aids in nutrient absorption, and promotes regular bowel movements. Aim to drink enough water throughout the day and listen to your body's hydration needs, especially during physical activity or in warm weather.

6. Practice Mindful Eating: Mindful eating is a practice that involves paying attention to the sensory experiences and cues of your eating experience. Slow down, savor your meals, and listen to your body's hunger and fullness cues. Chew your food thoroughly to aid in digestion and nutrient absorption. By practicing mindful eating, you can enhance digestion, reduce overeating, and foster a healthy relationship with food.

7. Seek Emotional Support: Emotional well-being is closely connected to gut health. Seek emotional support from friends, family, or professionals when needed. Engaging in activities that bring you joy, practicing self-care, and fostering healthy relationships can positively impact your gut and overall well-being.

Remember, restoring gut health is a journey, and the lifestyle modifications mentioned above should be implemented as part of a holistic approach. It's essential to listen to your body, be patient with the healing process, and work closely with healthcare professionals to address any underlying health conditions. By making these lifestyle modifications, you can create an environment that supports gut healing, promotes digestive wellness, and enhances your overall quality of life.

The Role of Probiotics and Prebiotics in Gut Restoration

Probiotics and prebiotics play vital roles in gut restoration by promoting a healthy gut microbiota, enhancing digestion, and supporting overall digestive wellness. Understanding the benefits and differences between probiotics and prebiotics can help you make informed choices to restore and maintain a healthy gut. Let's explore their roles in gut restoration:

Probiotics:
Probiotics are live bacteria or yeasts that provide numerous health benefits when consumed in adequate amounts. These beneficial microorganisms can help restore the balance of the gut microbiota, support digestion, and boost the immune system. Probiotics work by colonizing the gut, crowding out harmful bacteria, and producing compounds that promote gut health. They can also enhance the integrity

of the gut lining, reduce inflammation, and improve nutrient absorption.

Some common strains of probiotics include Lactobacillus acidophilus, Bifidobacterium lactis, and Saccharomyces boulardii. Probiotics can be found in various forms, including capsules, tablets, powders, and fermented foods. Incorporating probiotic-rich foods such as yogurt, kefir, sauerkraut, kimchi, and kombucha into your diet can introduce beneficial bacteria to support gut restoration.

Prebiotics:
Prebiotics, on the other hand, are non-digestible fibers that serve as food for beneficial bacteria in the gut. They act as a fuel source for probiotics and help them thrive and multiply. By selectively stimulating the growth and activity of beneficial bacteria, prebiotics contribute to a healthy gut microbiota and overall gut restoration.

Common sources of prebiotic fibers include chicory root, Jerusalem artichoke, onions, garlic, leeks, asparagus, bananas, and whole grains. Including these foods in your diet can provide the necessary prebiotic fibers to support gut health.

The Synergistic Relationship:
Probiotics and prebiotics work in synergy to promote gut restoration. While probiotics provide live beneficial bacteria, prebiotics serve as nourishment for these bacteria, helping them flourish and exert their beneficial effects. This symbiotic relationship between probiotics and prebiotics is known as synbiotics.

When taken together, probiotics and prebiotics can have a more significant impact on gut health compared to consuming them individually. Many products on the market combine probiotics and prebiotics to provide a synergistic effect.

Benefits of Probiotics and Prebiotics:
- Restoring and maintaining a healthy gut microbiota balance.
- Enhancing digestion and nutrient absorption.
- Supporting immune system function.
- Reducing inflammation in the gut.
- Alleviating symptoms of digestive disorders, such as bloating, gas, and diarrhea.
- Promoting regular bowel movements and relieving constipation.
- Supporting overall gut health and improving overall well-being.

It's important to note that the effectiveness of probiotics and prebiotics can vary based on individual needs and the specific strains and doses used. It's recommended to consult with a healthcare professional or a registered dietitian to determine the most appropriate probiotic and prebiotic supplements or dietary sources for your specific gut health goals.

In conclusion, probiotics and prebiotics play significant roles in gut restoration by supporting a healthy gut microbiota, improving digestion, and promoting overall digestive wellness. Incorporating probiotic-rich foods and prebiotic fibers into your diet can help restore balance in the gut and contribute to a healthy gut ecosystem. Consider incorporating these gut-friendly components as part of a comprehensive approach to gut restoration and overall well-being.

Chapter 6: Gut Health for the Whole Family: Supporting Children and Aging Adults

Nurturing a Healthy Gut from Early Childhood

The health of our gut begins early in life, and it is essential to prioritize the development and maintenance of a healthy gut microbiota from childhood. Early childhood is a critical period for gut health, as it can have a profound impact on long-term health outcomes, including digestion, immunity, and overall well-being. Here are some important factors to consider when nurturing a healthy gut in early childhood:

Breastfeeding:
Breast milk is nature's perfect food for infants, providing essential nutrients, antibodies, and a diverse array of beneficial bacteria. Breast milk contains prebiotics that

act as food for beneficial bacteria in the baby's gut, promoting the growth of a healthy gut microbiota. Breastfeeding for the recommended duration, typically at least six months, can have a positive impact on the development of the gut microbiota and support a healthy digestive system.

Introduction of Solid Foods:
When the time comes to introduce solid foods, it is important to focus on a diverse and nutritious diet. Introduce a variety of fruits, vegetables, whole grains, and lean proteins to provide a broad range of nutrients and prebiotic fibers. This diversity helps to cultivate a healthy gut microbiota and supports the development of a robust immune system. Avoiding processed foods, excessive sugar, and artificial additives is crucial in nurturing a healthy gut from early childhood.

Probiotic-Rich Foods:
Introducing age-appropriate probiotic-rich foods can contribute to the development of a healthy gut microbiota. Foods like yogurt, kefir, and fermented vegetables contain live beneficial bacteria that can populate the gut and support digestive health. However, it is important to consider age recommendations and consult with a pediatrician or healthcare professional when incorporating probiotics into an infant or child's diet.

Reducing Antibiotic Use:
While antibiotics are important for treating bacterial infections, they can also disrupt the natural balance of bacteria in the gut. Excessive or unnecessary use of antibiotics during early childhood can have long-term consequences for gut health. It is crucial to follow appropriate antibiotic use guidelines and discuss alternatives with a healthcare professional when appropriate.

Promoting Outdoor Play and Physical Activity:
Engaging in regular outdoor play and physical activity can have a positive impact on gut health. Exposure to diverse environments, such as nature and outdoor spaces, helps introduce beneficial microbes into the gut and supports the development of a diverse gut microbiota. Encouraging active play and spending time in nature can contribute to overall well-being and foster a healthy gut ecosystem.

Emphasizing Hygiene Practices:
While exposure to beneficial microbes is essential for gut health, it is equally important to maintain proper hygiene practices. Teaching children good hand-washing habits, especially before meals and after using the restroom, helps prevent the transmission of harmful bacteria that can disrupt gut health.

Creating a Healthy Food Environment:
Parents and caregivers play a crucial role in creating a healthy food environment that supports gut health. Offer a variety of nutrient-rich foods, involve children in meal planning and preparation, and model healthy eating habits. Creating a positive and enjoyable food environment helps foster a healthy relationship with food and supports gut health from an early age.

By focusing on these aspects of nurturing a healthy gut from early childhood, you can set the foundation for optimal gut health and overall well-being throughout a child's life. Remember, each child is unique, and it's important to consult with pediatricians or healthcare professionals for personalized guidance and recommendations to support the specific needs of your child's gut health.

Gut Health Considerations for Seniors
As we age, maintaining optimal gut health becomes increasingly important for overall

well-being and quality of life. The gut microbiota, digestive function, and nutrient absorption can undergo changes with age, which may impact gut health. Here are some key considerations for seniors to promote and maintain a healthy gut:

Dietary Fiber Intake:
Adequate dietary fiber intake is crucial for maintaining a healthy gut and supporting regular bowel movements. However, older adults often face challenges in meeting their fiber needs due to decreased appetite, dental issues, or digestive concerns. Including fiber-rich foods such as whole grains, fruits, vegetables, legumes, and nuts in the diet can help promote healthy digestion and provide essential nutrients. It is important to gradually increase fiber intake and stay hydrated to prevent discomfort or constipation.

Proper Hydration:
Maintaining proper hydration is essential for gut health, as it supports regular bowel movements and prevents constipation. Seniors may have reduced thirst sensations, making it important to consciously drink enough water throughout the day. Herbal teas, infused water, and hydrating foods like soups and fruits can also contribute to overall hydration.

Probiotics and Fermented Foods:
Including probiotics and fermented foods in the diet can support a healthy gut microbiota, which plays a crucial role in digestive function and immune health. Probiotics are beneficial bacteria that can be consumed through supplements or naturally found in fermented foods like yogurt, kefir, sauerkraut, and kimchi. These foods can help maintain a diverse gut microbiota and support optimal digestion.

Digestive Enzymes:
Seniors may experience a decline in the production of digestive enzymes, which are necessary for breaking down food and absorbing nutrients. This can lead to digestive discomfort and nutrient deficiencies. Consulting with a healthcare professional to assess the need for digestive enzyme supplements can help support digestion and nutrient absorption.

Medication Management:
Seniors often take multiple medications, which can have an impact on gut health. Some medications may disrupt the gut microbiota or cause digestive side effects. It is important to discuss any concerns or potential side effects with healthcare providers and explore strategies to minimize the impact on gut health, such as adjusting medication timing or considering alternative options.

Regular Physical Activity:
Engaging in regular physical activity can help promote healthy digestion and bowel regularity. Exercise stimulates the muscles of the gastrointestinal tract, aiding in the movement of food through the digestive system. It also supports overall well-being and can help manage stress, which can have an impact on gut health.

Stress Management:
Chronic stress can negatively affect gut health and digestive function. Seniors may face unique stressors, such as health concerns, lifestyle changes, or loss of loved ones. Implementing stress management techniques like mindfulness, meditation, deep breathing exercises, or engaging in enjoyable activities can support a healthy gut and overall well-being.

Regular Check-ups and Screenings:
Regular check-ups with healthcare providers are important for monitoring gut

health and identifying any potential issues. Screening for conditions such as colorectal cancer or gastrointestinal disorders should be part of routine healthcare for seniors. Early detection and intervention can help manage and prevent complications related to gut health.

In conclusion, seniors can support and maintain a healthy gut by focusing on dietary fiber intake, hydration, probiotics, digestive enzymes, medication management, regular physical activity, stress management, and regular check-ups. Consulting with healthcare professionals and registered dietitians who specialize in geriatric nutrition can provide personalized guidance and recommendations tailored to individual needs. Prioritizing gut health can contribute to overall well-being, digestive wellness, and a higher quality of life in the senior years.

Gut-Friendly Tips for the Whole Family
Maintaining a healthy gut is essential for the well-being of every family member. By adopting gut-friendly habits and making conscious choices about nutrition and lifestyle, you can support the health of your entire family. Here are some practical tips for cultivating a gut-friendly environment at home:

1. Embrace a Plant-Rich Diet: Incorporate a wide variety of fruits, vegetables, whole grains, legumes, and nuts into your family's meals. These fiber-rich foods provide nourishment for the beneficial bacteria in the gut and support a diverse gut microbiota.

2. Prioritize Probiotic Foods: Introduce probiotic-rich foods into your family's diet, such as yogurt, kefir, sauerkraut, kimchi, and other fermented foods. These foods contain live bacteria that can populate the gut and contribute to a healthy microbiome.

3. Limit Processed Foods and Added Sugars: Minimize the consumption of processed and packaged foods, as they often contain artificial additives, preservatives, and excessive amounts of added sugars. These can disrupt the balance of gut bacteria and contribute to digestive issues.

4. Encourage Hydration: Ensure that your family members stay adequately hydrated by drinking plenty of water throughout the day. Water supports healthy digestion, aids in nutrient absorption, and helps maintain regular bowel movements.

5. Practice Mindful Eating: Teach your family the importance of mindful eating. Encourage them to slow down, chew their food thoroughly, and savor each bite. This allows for better digestion and absorption of nutrients.

6. Cook and Prepare Meals Together: Involve your family in meal planning, grocery shopping, and cooking. This not only fosters a sense of togetherness but also encourages healthier food choices and the development of essential cooking skills.

7. Promote Regular Physical Activity: Engage in regular physical activities as a family, such as going for walks, bike rides, or playing outdoor games. Physical exercise stimulates the muscles of the digestive system and supports healthy bowel movements.

8. Manage Stress Levels: High levels of stress can negatively impact gut health. Encourage stress management techniques, such as deep breathing exercises, yoga, meditation, or engaging in hobbies and activities that promote relaxation and well-being.

9. Prioritize Sleep: Good quality sleep is essential for overall health, including gut health. Establish consistent sleep routines for family members and ensure they get the recommended amount of sleep for their age.

10. Create a Positive Food Environment: Foster a positive and supportive food environment at home. Avoid using food as a reward or punishment and encourage a balanced and intuitive approach to eating. Focus on nourishing the body with wholesome foods rather than restrictive diets or strict rules.

11. Practice Food Safety: Educate your family about proper food handling and food safety practices to prevent foodborne illnesses. Ensure that food is stored, prepared, and cooked safely to avoid contamination.

12. Regular Family Meals: Aim to have regular family meals together as often as

possible. Eating meals as a family encourages connection, communication, and the sharing of healthy eating habits.

By implementing these gut-friendly tips, you can promote the well-being of your entire family and cultivate a healthy gut environment for everyone. Remember, small changes over time can have a significant impact on gut health, leading to improved digestion, better nutrient absorption, and overall vitality for each family member.

Building Healthy Habits for Long-Term Gut Health

Achieving and maintaining optimal gut health requires the cultivation of healthy habits that support the well-being of your digestive system. By incorporating these habits into your daily routine, you can promote long-term gut health and overall vitality. Here are some key habits to consider:

1. Eat a Balanced Diet: Focus on consuming a balanced and varied diet that includes a wide range of nutrient-dense foods. Emphasize fruits, vegetables, whole grains, lean proteins, and healthy fats. This provides essential vitamins, minerals, fiber, and antioxidants that support a healthy gut and overall well-being.

2. Prioritize Fiber Intake: Increase your intake of dietary fiber, as it plays a crucial role in maintaining a healthy gut. Fiber-rich foods like fruits, vegetables, whole grains, legumes, and nuts promote regular bowel movements, support beneficial gut bacteria, and help prevent digestive issues.

3. Stay Hydrated: Drink an adequate amount of water throughout the day to support digestion and maintain optimal hydration. Water helps soften stools, aids in nutrient absorption, and facilitates the movement of waste through the digestive system.

4. Practice Portion Control: Be mindful of portion sizes and listen to your body's hunger and fullness cues. Overeating can put strain on the digestive system, leading to discomfort and digestive issues. Aim to eat until you are satisfied, not overly full.

5. Chew Your Food Thoroughly: Take the time to chew your food thoroughly before swallowing. Proper chewing aids in the breakdown of food and promotes better digestion. It also allows for the release of digestive enzymes in the mouth, which aids in nutrient absorption.

6. Minimize Processed Foods: Reduce your consumption of processed and packaged foods that are often high in added sugars, unhealthy fats, and artificial additives. These can disrupt the balance of gut bacteria and contribute to inflammation and digestive issues.

7. Include Fermented Foods: Incorporate fermented foods into your diet, such as yogurt, kefir, sauerkraut, kimchi, and kombucha. These foods contain beneficial bacteria that can help populate and diversify the gut microbiota, supporting a healthy gut environment.

8. Manage Stress Levels: Chronic stress can impact gut health by altering the gut-brain axis and contributing to digestive issues. Implement stress management techniques such as exercise, meditation, deep breathing, and engaging in activities that promote relaxation and well-being.

9. Regular Physical Activity: Engage in regular physical activity to support healthy digestion. Exercise stimulates the muscles of the gastrointestinal tract, promoting proper bowel movements and aiding in the elimination of waste.

10. Get Sufficient Sleep: Prioritize quality sleep to support overall health, including gut health. Aim for the recommended amount of sleep for your age group to allow for proper digestion and rejuvenation of the body.

11. Practice Good Hygiene: Maintain good hygiene practices, including washing your hands regularly, especially before meals, to prevent the spread of harmful bacteria that can disrupt gut health.

12. Limit Alcohol and Smoking: Excessive alcohol consumption and smoking can have a negative impact on gut health. Limit alcohol intake and avoid smoking to promote a healthy gut environment.

13. Regular Check-ups: Schedule regular check-ups with your healthcare provider to monitor your gut health and address any concerns or symptoms promptly. They can provide guidance tailored to your specific

needs and recommend appropriate tests if necessary.

Remember, building healthy habits takes time and consistency. Start by incorporating one or two habits at a time and gradually integrate more into your daily routine. By committing to these habits, you can promote long-term gut health and enjoy the benefits of a well-functioning digestive system, improved nutrient absorption, and overall well-being.

Chapter 7: Maintaining Gut Health in a Modern World

Navigating Gut Health Challenges in Our Environment

In today's modern world, our environment can pose various challenges to gut health. From exposure to pollutants and toxins to the prevalence of processed foods, it's important to be aware of these challenges and take proactive steps to mitigate their impact on our digestive system. Here are some key considerations and strategies for navigating gut health challenges in our environment:

1. Environmental Toxins: Our environment is filled with toxins that can have detrimental effects on gut health. Pesticides, heavy metals, air pollutants, and chemicals found in household products can disrupt the delicate balance of the gut microbiota and contribute to inflammation and digestive issues. Minimize exposure to toxins by

choosing organic produce, using natural cleaning products, and reducing exposure to pollutants whenever possible.

2. Food Quality: The quality of our food has a direct impact on gut health. Processed foods, artificial additives, preservatives, and excessive amounts of added sugars can disrupt the balance of gut bacteria and contribute to inflammation. Opt for whole, unprocessed foods as much as possible, and prioritize organic and locally sourced options to minimize exposure to pesticides and other contaminants.

3. Antibiotic Use: Antibiotics can be lifesaving in certain situations, but they can also disrupt the gut microbiota by indiscriminately killing off both harmful and beneficial bacteria. If you require antibiotics, discuss with your healthcare provider about strategies to mitigate their impact on gut health, such as probiotic supplementation or

taking prebiotic-rich foods to support the growth of beneficial bacteria.

4. Stress and Lifestyle Factors: Chronic stress, inadequate sleep, and sedentary lifestyles can all impact gut health. Stress affects the gut-brain axis, leading to digestive issues, while lack of sleep and physical inactivity can slow down digestion and contribute to constipation. Prioritize stress management techniques, get sufficient sleep, and engage in regular physical activity to support a healthy gut environment.

5. Gut-disruptive Medications: Certain medications, such as nonsteroidal anti-inflammatory drugs (NSAIDs), proton pump inhibitors (PPIs), and oral contraceptives, can have an impact on gut health. These medications may increase the risk of gastrointestinal issues like gut inflammation, altered gut microbiota, and increased intestinal permeability. If you are

on long-term medication, discuss potential gut health side effects with your healthcare provider and explore ways to minimize their impact through lifestyle modifications or alternative treatment options.

6. Hydration and Water Quality: Proper hydration is crucial for maintaining healthy digestion. Ensure that you drink clean, filtered water to avoid contaminants that can affect gut health. In regions where water quality is a concern, consider investing in a reliable water filtration system or drinking bottled water from trusted sources.

7. Food Sensitivities and Allergies: Food sensitivities and allergies can cause gut inflammation and digestive distress. Identify and manage any food sensitivities or allergies by working with a healthcare provider or a registered dietitian who can guide you through an elimination diet or other appropriate testing methods.

8. Environmental Allergens: Allergens present in the environment, such as pollen, dust mites, and pet dander, can trigger allergic reactions and cause gut-related symptoms like bloating, diarrhea, or constipation. Minimize exposure to allergens through proper home cleaning, air filtration systems, and allergy management strategies.

9. Digestive Disorders and Diseases: Individuals with specific digestive disorders or diseases, such as irritable bowel syndrome (IBS), inflammatory bowel disease (IBD), or celiac disease, face unique challenges in maintaining gut health. Work closely with healthcare professionals to manage and treat these conditions through personalized dietary and lifestyle interventions.

10. Gut-Supportive Practices: Incorporate gut-supportive practices into your daily routine to counterbalance environmental

challenges. These practices may include consuming a nutrient

-dense diet, taking appropriate supplements under professional guidance, practicing stress management techniques, getting regular exercise, and engaging in activities that promote relaxation and well-being.

By understanding and addressing the gut health challenges present in our environment, we can take proactive steps to support and optimize our digestive well-being. Remember, everyone's journey to gut health is unique, so it's important to listen to your body, work with qualified healthcare professionals, and make choices that align with your individual needs and circumstances.

Strategies for Managing Gut Health While Traveling

Traveling can be an exciting and enriching experience, but it can also disrupt your gut health routine. Changes in diet, water quality, time zone differences, and stress levels can all affect your digestive system. However, with a little preparation and mindful choices, you can manage and support your gut health while traveling. Here are some strategies to consider:

1. Plan Ahead: Research your travel destination to familiarize yourself with the local cuisine and food options. Look for restaurants that offer fresh, whole foods and prioritize hygiene practices. Consider packing some gut-friendly snacks, such as nuts, seeds, or dried fruits, to have on hand during your journey.

2. Stay Hydrated: Proper hydration is essential for maintaining a healthy digestive system. Carry a refillable water bottle and drink plenty of water throughout your trip. If you are uncertain about the quality of tap water at your destination, opt for bottled water or use a water purifier.

3. Be Mindful of Food Choices: While traveling, it's tempting to indulge in new and exotic foods. However, pay attention to your body's cues and make mindful food choices. Opt for balanced meals that include vegetables, lean proteins, and whole grains. Be cautious of street food and ensure that it is prepared in hygienic conditions.

4. Pack Digestive Support: Consider bringing digestive aids such as probiotics or digestive enzymes to support your gut health during travel. Consult with a healthcare professional to determine the appropriate supplements for your needs.

5. Practice Portion Control: It can be easy to overeat while on vacation, but overindulging can strain your digestive system. Practice portion control and listen to your body's signals of fullness.

6. Maintain Regular Meal Times: Try to stick to a regular eating schedule as much as possible, even if it means adjusting to a different time zone. Consistency in meal times helps regulate your digestion and minimize potential disruptions.

7. Avoid Excessive Alcohol and Caffeine: Both alcohol and caffeine can disrupt gut health and contribute to digestive issues. Limit your consumption of these substances, especially if you are prone to digestive sensitivities.

8. Stay Active: Physical activity supports healthy digestion, so find ways to incorporate movement into your travel routine. Explore the local area on foot, take a yoga class, or simply stretch and move your body regularly.

9. Manage Stress: Traveling can be stressful, which can impact your gut health. Implement stress management techniques

such as deep breathing, meditation, or engaging in activities that help you relax and unwind.

10. Rest and Sleep: Proper rest and sufficient sleep are essential for gut health. Prioritize sleep and establish a bedtime routine, even while traveling. Create a comfortable sleep environment to support your body's natural rhythms.

11. Wash Your Hands: Good hygiene practices, such as washing your hands regularly, can help prevent the spread of harmful bacteria and reduce the risk of gastrointestinal infections.

12. Be Mindful of Traveler's Diarrhea: Traveler's diarrhea can be a common occurrence when visiting certain destinations. Be cautious of uncooked or undercooked foods, drink bottled or filtered water, and avoid ice cubes made from tap water.

13. Listen to Your Body: Pay attention to any digestive discomfort or changes in bowel movements while traveling. If you experience persistent symptoms or concerns, seek medical attention at your travel destination.

By implementing these strategies, you can support your gut health while enjoying your travel experiences. Remember that everyone's digestive system is unique, so be mindful of your individual needs and make choices that align with maintaining a healthy gut while exploring the world.

Balancing Gut Health in a Digital Age

In today's digital age, technology has become an integral part of our lives. While it offers numerous benefits and conveniences, it can also have implications for our gut health. The constant exposure to screens, sedentary lifestyles, and increased stress levels can all impact our digestive system.

However, with awareness and intentional practices, we can strive to balance our gut health in the midst of a digital world. Here are some strategies to consider:

1. Limit Screen Time: Excessive screen time can disrupt our eating habits and lead to mindless eating. Set boundaries for yourself by scheduling designated screen-free times or areas, especially during meals. This allows you to focus on your food, eat mindfully, and promote better digestion.

2. Practice Digital Detoxes: Take regular breaks from digital devices to give your body and mind a rest. Engage in activities that promote relaxation, such as reading a book, going for a walk in nature, or spending quality time with loved ones. Disconnecting from technology allows you to reduce stress levels and support overall well-being, including gut health.

3. Promote Physical Activity: The sedentary nature of digital lifestyles can contribute to sluggish digestion. Make a conscious effort to incorporate physical activity into your daily routine. Whether it's going for a walk, practicing yoga, or engaging in a favorite sport, movement helps stimulate digestion and supports a healthy gut.

4. Mindful Eating in a Digital World: Eating while distracted by screens can disrupt the digestive process. Practice mindful eating by being fully present and savoring each bite. Engage your senses, appreciate the flavors and textures of your food, and chew slowly. This allows for proper digestion and absorption of nutrients.

5. Prioritize Sleep: The blue light emitted by electronic devices can interfere with sleep quality. Establish a digital curfew by powering down devices at least an hour before bedtime. Create a relaxing bedtime routine to promote restful sleep, as quality

sleep is crucial for gut health and overall well-being.

6. Manage Stress: The constant connectivity and information overload of the digital world can contribute to increased stress levels. Chronic stress can disrupt gut health and contribute to digestive issues. Incorporate stress management techniques such as meditation, deep breathing exercises, or engaging in hobbies that bring you joy and relaxation.

7. Cultivate Healthy Relationships: While digital connections can be valuable, nurturing real-life relationships is equally important. Make time for face-to-face interactions with family and friends. Engaging in meaningful social connections promotes emotional well-being, reduces stress, and positively influences gut health.

8. Seek Balance in Online Information: The abundance of health information available

online can be overwhelming. Be discerning about the sources you rely on and consult trusted healthcare professionals for personalized guidance. Avoid falling into the trap of excessive self-diagnosis and self-treatment, as it can lead to unnecessary stress and potentially harm gut health.

9. Hydration and Gut Health: Digital distractions can sometimes lead to neglecting our hydration needs. Stay mindful of your water intake and aim to drink enough water throughout the day. Proper hydration supports digestion, helps maintain healthy bowel movements, and promotes a thriving gut environment.

10. Gut-Friendly Technology: While technology can impact gut health, it can also be a tool for supporting it. Utilize apps and wearable devices that promote mindfulness, track hydration, encourage physical activity, and provide guidance for healthy eating habits. Choose technology that aligns with

your well-being goals and helps you maintain a balanced approach to gut health.

By consciously balancing our digital lives with healthy lifestyle choices, we can support our gut health in the midst of a technology-driven world. Remember to listen to your body, cultivate awareness, and make choices that prioritize your overall well-being. Strive for a harmonious relationship with technology that allows you to nurture your gut health and thrive in the digital age.

Sustaining Gut-Friendly Practices for Lifelong Well-Being

Maintaining a healthy gut is not just a temporary endeavor—it is a lifelong commitment to your overall well-being. By adopting and sustaining gut-friendly practices, you can promote optimal digestive health and enjoy the benefits for years to come. Here are some key strategies to help you sustain a healthy gut for lifelong well-being:

1. Consistency is Key: Consistency is crucial when it comes to gut health. Aim to incorporate gut-friendly practices into your daily routine and make them a priority. Whether it's eating a balanced diet, staying hydrated, practicing stress management techniques, or engaging in regular physical activity, consistency will yield long-term benefits for your digestive system.

2. Mindful Eating: Practice mindful eating as a lifelong habit. Be aware of your food choices, eat slowly, chew thoroughly, and pay attention to your body's hunger and fullness cues. This allows you to optimize digestion, absorb nutrients effectively, and maintain a healthy gut environment.

3. Nourishing Diet: Adopt a nourishing and varied diet that includes a wide range of whole, unprocessed foods. Prioritize

fiber-rich fruits, vegetables, whole grains, legumes, and lean proteins. These foods provide essential nutrients and support a diverse gut microbiota, promoting long-term gut health.

4. Hydration Habits: Maintain healthy hydration habits by drinking an adequate amount of water throughout the day. Staying hydrated supports optimal digestion, aids in the elimination of waste, and helps maintain a healthy gut environment.

5. Regular Physical Activity: Incorporate regular physical activity into your daily life. Engaging in moderate exercise, such as walking, swimming, cycling, or practicing yoga, supports healthy digestion, promotes bowel regularity, and enhances overall well-being.

6. Stress Management: Chronic stress can negatively impact gut health. Implement stress management techniques that work for

you, such as meditation, deep breathing exercises, yoga, or engaging in hobbies that bring joy and relaxation. Cultivate a balanced lifestyle that prioritizes mental and emotional well-being.

7. Sleep Quality: Aim for restful and sufficient sleep each night. Quality sleep allows your body to repair and rejuvenate, which positively impacts gut health. Establish a regular sleep routine, create a comfortable sleep environment, and prioritize sleep as an integral part of your overall well-being.

8. Regular Check-Ups: Schedule regular check-ups with your healthcare provider to monitor your gut health and address any potential concerns. Regular screenings and assessments can help detect and manage any underlying conditions or imbalances before they become more significant issues.

9. Listen to Your Body: Tune in to your body's signals and listen to its needs. Pay attention to any changes in your digestion, bowel movements, or overall well-being. If you notice persistent symptoms or concerns, seek professional guidance to address them promptly.

10. Continuous Learning: Stay informed about the latest research and developments in gut health. Be open to learning and adapting your habits based on new information. Stay connected with reputable sources of information and consult with healthcare professionals to stay up to date on best practices for gut health.

11. Supportive Community: Surround yourself with a supportive community that values and prioritizes gut health. Engage in conversations, join online communities, or attend events where you can share experiences, exchange knowledge, and receive support on your gut health journey.

12. Adaptation and Flexibility: Remember that everyone's gut health journey is unique. Be open to adaptation and flexibility as you discover what works best for your body. Recognize that needs may change over time, and be willing to adjust your habits and practices accordingly.

By incorporating these strategies into your daily life and committing to sustaining gut-friendly practices, you can cultivate lifelong well-being and enjoy the benefits of a healthy gut for years to come. Embrace the journey of nourishing your gut, and let it be a cornerstone of your overall health and vitality.

Conclusion: Embracing a Vibrantly Healthy Gut

Congratulations on completing this journey towards understanding and nurturing your gut health! You have equipped yourself with valuable knowledge, practical strategies, and a deep appreciation for the vital role your gut plays in your overall well-being. Now, it's time to embrace a vibrantly healthy gut and reap the rewards of your efforts.

As you reflect on the insights gained throughout this book, remember that your gut health is not an isolated aspect of your well-being. It is intricately connected to your immune system, mental health, energy levels, and overall vitality. By prioritizing your gut health, you are taking a proactive step towards a healthier, happier, and more fulfilling life.

Embracing a vibrantly healthy gut starts with a mindset shift. It's about recognizing that you have the power to make choices that support your gut's optimal functioning. It's about listening to your body, cultivating self-awareness, and making conscious decisions that honor your unique needs.

Remember, this is not a quick fix or a one-time endeavor. It's a lifelong commitment to your well-being. Embrace the journey of self-discovery, experimentation, and growth as you continue to refine your gut-friendly habits and adapt them to different stages of life.

One of the most beautiful aspects of nurturing your gut is the ripple effect it can have on other areas of your life. When your gut is balanced and thriving, you may notice increased energy, mental clarity, improved mood, better digestion, and enhanced overall vitality. These positive changes can positively impact your relationships, work, and overall sense of fulfillment.

As you move forward, let your gut health journey be a catalyst for continued growth and transformation. Stay curious and open to new research, emerging practices, and evolving knowledge about gut health. Explore new recipes, try different gut-friendly foods, and share your experiences with others. Engage in conversations, build connections, and support those around you who are also on their own gut health journeys.

Remember to be kind to yourself along the way. Each person's journey is unique, and progress may come in different forms and at different paces. Celebrate the small victories, and don't be discouraged by setbacks. Embrace the process and trust that your commitment to nurturing your gut will yield long-lasting benefits.

In closing, I invite you to embark on this next chapter of your life with a renewed sense of purpose and a deep appreciation for the power of a vibrantly healthy gut. Embrace the joy of nourishing your body from within, and let it radiate through every aspect of your life.

Remember, you have the ability to cultivate a vibrantly healthy gut and enjoy the countless rewards it brings. So, take the knowledge you have gained, the strategies you have learned, and the inspiration within your heart, and embark on a journey of lifelong gut health, vitality, and well-being.

Your vibrant gut awaits.

www.ingramcontent.com/pod-product-compliance
Lightning Source LLC
Chambersburg PA
CBHW061646250726
48659CB00004B/1390